SBAs and EMQs in Paediatrics
for Medical Students

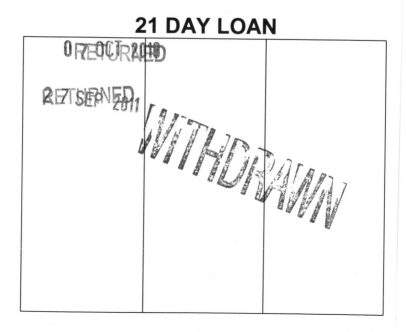

SBAs and EMQs in Paediatrics for Medical Students

DR NEEL SHARMA

BSc (Hons), MBChB
Foundation Year Two Doctor
Homerton University Hospital NHS Foundation Trust
London

Foreword by

DR TIAGO VILLANUEVA
Past Editor of the *Student BMJ*

Radcliffe Publishing
Oxford • New York

Radcliffe Publishing Ltd
18 Marcham Road
Abingdon
Oxon OX14 1AA
United Kingdom

www.radcliffe-oxford.com

Electronic catalogue and worldwide online ordering facility.

British Library Cataloguing in Publication Data

A catalogue record for this book is available from the British Library.

ISBN-13: 978 184619 429 0

The paper used for the text pages of this book is FSC certified. FSC (The Forest Stewardship Council) is an international network to promote responsible management of the world's forests.

Mixed Sources
Product group from well-managed
forests and other controlled sources
www.fsc.org Cert no. SGS-COC-2482
© 1996 Forest Stewardship Council

FSC

Typeset by Pindar NZ, Auckland, New Zealand
Printed and bound by TJI Digital, Padstow, Cornwall, UK

Contents

Foreword

Paediatrics is one of the most challenging fields in medicine. Whether you're a medical student just starting out on your clinical rotations and looking to grasp the initial concepts of paediatrics, or a final year student revising for your degree-qualifying exams, Dr Neel Sharma's new paediatrics SBA and EMQ book will certainly benefit your professional development.

Neel Sharma's SBAs and EMQs simulate many common and not-so-common clinical scenarios, which students are guaranteed to find in both the hospital and primary care setting. In my opinion, this will apply not only to home-grown students but also to students based outside the UK.

Dr Sharma has definitely mastered the art of producing a comprehensive, evidence-based review tool of core paediatric knowledge, while at the same time appealing to a broad audience, which in my opinion is quite a remarkable achievement. You're definitely looking at an invaluable resource, and buying this book will help you to rise up to the challenge that is the complexity of paediatrics.

Dr Tiago Villanueva
Past Editor of the *Student BMJ*
November 2009

Preface

As a recent medical graduate I understand all too well the pressures faced during medical school. Lectures, tutorials, never-ending ward rounds, outpatient clinics, course work assignments and, of course, let us not forget the gruelling end-of-year exams. Trying to retain and, more importantly, understand all the common (and not-so-common) clinical diseases and presentations truly seems an impossible task.

With the advent of the Universities Medical Assessment Partnership (UMAP) there has now been a move away from testing specific clinical facts to an assessment focused on preparing yourself as a foundation doctor and the knowledge such a trainee needs on a daily basis. Currently, 14 UK medical schools are part of UMAP and their exams now require candidates to decide, for example, what would be the most appropriate initial investigation or what management plan they would instigate first when faced with a clinical problem – hardly an easy task based on the little experience one gains as an undergraduate in such decisions.

This self-assessment book is designed to help students tackle both the new form of assessment as well as the traditional style of examination. Questions covering all common paediatric presentations are included as SBA and EMQ formats with relevant, concise explanations as answers.

I sincerely hope that this book is of use in preparing for your forthcoming examinations and wish you all the success in your future medical careers.

Neel Sharma
November 2009

Education and work are the levers to uplift a people. Work alone will not do it unless inspired by the right ideals and guided by intelligence.

WEB Du Bois 1868–1963

I would like to dedicate this book to my parents, Ravi and Anita, and my sister Ravnita. Without their continued support and encouragement none of this would have truly been possible.

Useful references

Journal of Pediatrics. Available at: www.jpeds.com

Journal of Paediatrics and Child Health. Available at: www.wiley.com/bw/journal.asp?ref=1034–4810

Tasker R, McClure R, Acerini C. *Oxford Handbook of Paediatrics*. Oxford: Oxford University Press; 2008.

The Royal College of Paediatrics and Child Health. Available at: www.rcpch.ac.uk

Questions

Single best answer

1   A mother brings her two-month-old baby to the GP for a routine check up. The following motor milestones are all commonly observed at this age EXCEPT:

    a   The grasp reflex

    b   The moro reflex

    c   The rooting reflex

    d   The pacing reflex

    e   Palmar grasp

2   What is the most likely time frame when the primitive reflexes disappear?

    a   Birth

    b   1 month

    c   40 weeks

    d   3 to 9 months

    e   2 months

3   The following statements are all true for children at six months of
    age EXCEPT:

    a   They can be pulled to sit with a straight back

    b   They can kick their legs

    c   They can demonstrate a palmar grasp

    d   They can no longer demonstrate the primitive reflexes

    e   They can crawl

4   The following motor milestones are all commonly observed bet-
    ween the ages of 9 and 15 months EXCEPT:

    a   Sitting unsupported

    b   Walking

    c   Bottom shuffling

    d   Being pulled to stand

    e   Pincer grip

5   The following motor milestones are all commonly observed bet-
    ween the ages of 18 and 30 months EXCEPT:

    a   Walking

    b   Climbing onto furniture

    c   Jumping

    d   Running

    e   Dressing

6 The following motor milestones are all commonly observed between the ages of 36 and 48 months EXCEPT:

a Dressing

b Hand dominance

c Jumping

d Throwing a ball

e Drawing a person with a head

7 The following communication skills are all commonly observed between the ages of 12 and 24 months EXCEPT:

a Babbling

b Following a simple command

c Repetition of words

d Use of words with meaning

e Repetition of phrases

8 A four-year-old boy is brought to his GP by his mother. She is concerned that he is unable to dress by himself and do simple tasks such as drawing and playing with a ball. What is the most likely diagnosis?

a Mental retardation

b Dyspraxia

c Dyslexia

d Ataxia

e None of the above

9 A six-year-old boy is brought to his GP by his father. His father is concerned that his son is wetting the bed at night. His father himself had a history of nocturnal enuresis as a child. The boy appears otherwise well. Routine observations are within normal limits for his age. What is the next most appropriate initial investigation?

a Urine dipstick

b Renal ultrasound scan

c Abdominal X-ray

d Computed tomography (CT) scan lumbar spine

e Urine microscopy and culture

10 What is the next most appropriate step in management in the above case?

a Desmopressin (DDAVP)

b Enuresis alarm

c Continue to observe

d Demeclocycline

e Star chart

11 A six-year-old boy is brought to his GP by his mother. His mother is noted to be low in mood, tearful and withdrawn. She comments that she can no longer cope with life and feels like a bad mother. During the consultation you observe bruises on the boy's face and neck. On further inspection you note the bruises are 'finger tip' shaped. What is the next most appropriate step in management?

   a Call the police

   b Continue to observe

   c Urgent international normalised ratio (INR) and liver function tests

   d Liaise with social services

   e Section the mother

12 A newborn baby boy is assessed by the on-call paediatrician. On examination he notes a rigid foot posture that proves difficult to correct. What is the most likely diagnosis?

   a Hammer foot

   b Talipes equinovarus

   c Genu varum

   d Genu valgum

   e Pigeon toe

13 A two-year-old boy is brought to his GP by his mother. She is concerned about his walking ability. On assessment of his gait you observe bowing of the tibia and inwardly turned ankle joints. What is the most likely diagnosis?

   a Hammer foot

   b Talipes equinovarus

   c Genu varum

   d Genu valgum

   e Pigeon toe

14 A five-year-old girl is brought to A&E by her mother. She is concerned about her daughter's ability to walk. On gait assessment you note that her knees are held together with her ankles placed wide apart. What is the most likely diagnosis?

   a Hammer foot

   b Talipes equinovarus

   c Genu varum

   d Genu valgum

   e Pigeon toe

15 A boy was recently diagnosed with pes planus. What other abnormality is he most likely to demonstrate?

   a Hammer foot

   b Talipes equinovarus

   c Genu varum

   d Genu valgum

   e Pigeon toe

16 An eight-year-old boy is brought to A&E by his mother. He complains of severe pain in his right hip, which radiates to his knee. His mother comments that he has recently suffered from a cold. On examination there is evidence of limited right hip movement. Routine observations demonstrate a temperature of 38°C. What is the most likely diagnosis?

a Transient synovitis of the hip

b Legg Calve Perthes disease

c Slipped upper femoral epiphysis

d Developmental dysplasia of the hip

e Septic arthritis

17 A boy is recently diagnosed with transient synovitis of the hip. Which management plan would you instigate first?

a Non-steroidal anti-inflammatory drugs (NSAIDs)

b Surgery

c Morphine

d Fentanyl patch

e Reassure

18 A boy is recently diagnosed with transient synovitis of the hip. What type of hip movement is most likely to be reduced?

a Flexion

b Extension

c Internal rotation

d External rotation

e Abduction

19 A 10-year-old boy is brought to A&E with a limp. On examination you note evidence of limb shortening. A lower limb X-ray demonstrates increased density in the femoral epiphysis bilaterally. What is the most likely diagnosis?

a Transient synovitis of the hip

b Legg Calve Perthes disease

c Slipped upper femoral epiphysis

d Developmental dysplasia of the hip

e Septic arthritis

20 What is the next most appropriate step in management of the above patient?

a Morphine

b Continue to observe

c Surgery

d Traction

e NSAIDs

21 An 11-year-old boy presents to A&E with a limp. On examination you observe evidence of reduced abduction and internal rotation. What is the most likely diagnosis?

a Transient synovitis of the hip

b Legg Calve Perthes disease

c Slipped upper femoral epiphysis

d Developmental dysplasia of the hip

e Septic arthritis

22 What is the next most appropriate initial investigation in the above patient?

    a Blood cultures

    b X-ray

    c Magnetic Resonance Imaging (MRI) scan

    d Ultrasound scan

    e Joint aspiration

23 A newborn baby is undergoing routine assessment. The paediatrician abducts one hip at a time in flexion while applying anterior pressure to the greater trochanter. He notes that there is absence of a 'clunk' felt as the hip relocates from this position. What is the most likely diagnosis?

    a Transient synovitis of the hip

    b Legg Calve Perthes disease

    c Slipped upper femoral epiphysis

    d Developmental dysplasia of the hip

    e Septic arthritis

24 What is the next most appropriate initial investigation in the above patient?

    a Ultrasound

    b X-ray

    c MRI scan

    d CT scan

    e Joint aspiration

25 A one-year-old boy is brought to A&E by his mother. The mother notes that he has been crying excessively and appears in severe pain. On examination you note evidence of rigid limbs. Routine blood investigations demonstrate a white cell count of 14×10^9/L and a C reactive protein of 85 mg/L. What is the most likely diagnosis?

    a Transient synovitis of the hip

    b Legg Calve Perthes disease

    c Slipped upper femoral epiphysis

    d Developmental dysplasia of the hip

    e Septic arthritis

26 A mother brings her son to A&E. He complains of sudden onset pain in his right leg. Routine observations demonstrate a temperature of 39°C. On examination you note tenderness on palpation with swelling and erythema. He refuses to weight bear. What is the most likely diagnosis?

    a Transient synovitis of the hip

    b Legg Calve Perthes disease

    c Osteomyelitis

    d Developmental dysplasia of the hip

    e Septic arthritis

27 What is the most likely aetiological cause for the above patient's symptoms?

    a *Staphylococcus aureus*

    b *Salmonella*

    c *Haemophilus influenzae*

    d *Streptococcus pyogenes*

    e *Mycobacterium tuberculosis*

28 A nine-year-boy is diagnosed with osteomyelitis. Which management plan would you instigate first?

   a Flucloxacillin

   b Morphine

   c Fentanyl patch

   d Aspirin

   e Rifampicin

29 A 10-year-old girl has been reviewed in A&E with a painful right limb. A diagnosis of osteomyelitis is suspected and an X-ray is ordered. What is most likely to be seen on the X-ray?

   a Hot spots

   b Osteophytes

   c Subperiosteal bone formation

   d Hairline fracture

   e Pepper pot appearance

30 A two-year-old boy is reviewed by his GP with his mother. He has recently been diagnosed with osteomyelitis for which he received antibiotics. On examination you note evidence of a severely swollen right knee, which is painful and warm to touch. What is the most likely diagnosis?

   a Transient synovitis of the hip

   b Legg Calve Perthes disease

   c Slipped upper femoral epiphysis

   d Developmental dysplasia of the hip

   e Septic arthritis

31 A 10-year-old girl is brought to her GP by her mother. Her mother is concerned about new onset swelling of her daughter's hands. On examination you note swelling of her metacarpophalangeal and proximal interphalangeal joints. What is the next most appropriate step in management?

a Paracetamol

b Morphine

c Reassure

d NSAIDs

e Methotrexate

32 A seven-year-old boy is brought to his GP by his mother. He has recently suffered a cold. His mother is concerned about the presence of a rash on his arms, legs and buttocks. On examination you note the presence of a maculopapular non-blanching rash. Routine observations reveal a temperature of 39°C. She also comments that when he opens his bowels his stool is tar-like in appearance. What is the most likely diagnosis?

a Gastritis

b Duodenal ulcer

c Meningitis

d Henoch Schonlein purpura

e Eczema

33 A newborn baby boy develops jaundice within 24 hours of birth. Which management plan would you instigate first?

a Phototherapy

b Liver ultrasound scan

c Abdominal X-ray

d Liver function tests

e Observe

34 A six-year-old boy is taken to A&E. He is pale and jaundiced in appearance. Routine blood investigations demonstrate a haemoglobin of 6 g/dL. A blood film is requested which indicates the presence of 'golf balls' following appropriate staining. What is the most likely diagnosis?

a Spherocytosis

b Thalassaemia

c Iron deficiency anaemia

d Sickle cell disease

e Vitamin B12 deficiency

35 A seven-year-old Indian boy is diagnosed with a form of anaemia. On examination you note evidence of frontal bossing. What is the most likely diagnosis?

a Spherocytosis

b Alpha thalassaemia

c Beta thalassaemia

d Delta thalassaemia

e Sickle cell disease

36   A four-year-old boy is brought to A&E by his mother following a fall. On examination you note a small cut on his knee that is failing to stop bleeding. Investigations confirm a diagnosis of haemophilia A. What is the next most appropriate step in management?

a Factor VIII

b Factor IX

c Mefenamic acid

d Tranexamic acid

e Aspirin

37   A five-year-old girl is brought to A&E following a nose bleed. She has recently suffered a viral infection. On examination you note evidence of generalised bruising. Routine investigations demonstrate a haemoglobin of 14 g/dL, a platelet count of 60×10^9/L, normal liver function tests and an INR of less than 1. What is the most likely diagnosis?

a Haemophilia A

b Haemophilia B

c Autoimmune thrombocytopenic purpura

d Von Willebrand's disease

e Disseminated intravascular coagulation

38   Which management plan would you instigate first in the above patient?

a Factor VIII

b Factor IX

c Mefenamic acid

d Tranexamic acid

e Platelet transfusion

39 A child is diagnosed with haemophilia B. What is the next most appropriate step in management?

a Factor VIII

b Factor IX

c Mefenamic acid

d Tranexamic acid

e Platelet transfusion

40 A seven-year-old boy is brought to A&E by his mother. She is concerned about his experience of continuous nose bleeds. Investigations demonstrate an activated partial thromboplastin time (APTT) of 40 seconds, a bleeding time of 12 minutes and a platelet count of 300×10^9/L. What is the most likely diagnosis?

a Haemophilia A

b Haemophilia B

c Autoimmune thrombocytopenic purpura

d Von Willebrand's disease

e Disseminated intravascular coagulation

41 A young girl is diagnosed with von Willebrand's disease. What additional clotting factor is most likely to be deficient?

a Factor VIII

b Factor V

c Factor IX

d Factor VI

e Factor VII

42 An eight-year-old boy is diagnosed with von Willebrand's disease. What is the next most appropriate step in management?

a Factor VII

b Factor IX

c Mefenamic acid

d Desmopressin (DDAVP)

e Platelet transfusion

43 A 12-year-old girl presents to her GP with her mother. She has been experiencing nose bleeds and bleeding of her gums. On further inspection you note evidence of oral candida. Blood investigations demonstrate a haemoglobin of 7 g/dL, a white cell count of 2 × 10^9/L and a platelet count of 25 × 10^9/L. What is the most likely diagnosis?

a Aplastic anaemia

b Thalassaemia

c G6PD deficiency

d Leukaemia

e Von Willebrand's disease

44 What investigation is most likely to confirm a diagnosis in the above patient?

a Bone marrow examination

b Reticulocyte count

c Mean corpuscular volume (MCV)

d Serum bilirubin

e Neutrophil count

45 A six-year-old boy is brought to A&E by his mother. He has been suffering from a sore throat and chesty cough for the past two weeks. On examination you note evidence of non-specific bruises and pallor. Blood investigations demonstrate a haemoglobin of 6 g/dL, a white cell count of 100×10^9/L and a platelet count of 50×10^9/L. A blood film demonstrates evidence of blast cells. What is the most likely diagnosis?

a Aplastic anaemia

b Hodgkin's lymphoma

c Chronic myeloid leukaemia

d Acute leukaemia

e Chronic lymphoblastic leukaemia

46 A five-year-old boy is diagnosed with leukaemia and subsequently commenced on treatment. The haematologist in charge of his care is concerned about the possibility of acute tumour lysis syndrome. The following are all features of acute tumour lysis syndrome EXCEPT:

a Hypokalemia

b Hyperuricemia

c Hyperphosphatemia

d Hypocalcaemia

e Elevated serum urea

47   A six-year-old boy is brought to his GP following concerns raised by his mother. His mother comments that he has developed a swelling on the right side of his neck. He has recently been suffering from a viral infection. On examination you note evidence of submandibular and supraclavicular lymphadenopathy. Routine observations demonstrate a temperature of 37°C. He appears otherwise well. What is the most likely aetiological cause for this presentation?

   a *Streptococcus*

   b *Haemophilus influenzae*

   c *Mycobacterium tuberculosis*

   d *Mycoplasma pneumoniae*

   e *Legionella*

48   An eight-year-old boy is seen in A&E accompanied by his father. His father is concerned about the fact that his son has been experiencing night sweats and a fever on and off. On examination you note the presence of firm painless swellings of his cervical lymph nodes. You arrange an urgent biopsy. Histology confirms the presence of Reed-Sternberg cells. What is the most likely diagnosis?

   a Non-Hodgkin's lymphoma

   b Hodgkin's lymphoma

   c Acute myeloid leukaemia

   d Acute lymphoblastic leukaemia

   e Chronic lymphoblastic leukaemia

49 Which of the following accounts for half of all brain tumours in children and arises from astrocytes?

a Medulloblastoma

b Glioma

c Neuroblastoma

d Wilm's tumour

e Craniopharyngioma

50 Which of the following brain tumours in children is a benign tumour associated with solid and cystic elements with calcification?

a Medulloblastoma

b Glioma

c Neuroblastoma

d Wilm's tumour

e Craniopharyngioma

51 A five-year-old boy is brought to A&E. His mother is deeply concerned as she has noticed that her son's eye movements appear jerky as if they are dancing. On examination the boy appears cachectic. He is below the normal range in terms of height and weight for his centile. What is the most likely diagnosis?

a Medulloblastoma

b Glioma

c Neuroblastoma

d Wilm's tumour

e Craniopharyngioma

52 What is the next most appropriate initial investigation for the above patient?

  a Urinary catecholamines

  b Full blood count

  c Serum cholesterol

  d Optometry assessment

  e Serum CA 19–9

53 A boy is recently diagnosed with neuroblastoma. What additional manifestation is he most likely to demonstrate on examination?

  a Ataxia

  b Abdominal mass

  c Upgoing plantars

  d Dysdiadokokinesis

  e Hypotonia

54 A seven-year-old girl is diagnosed with a Wilm's tumour following an abdominal ultrasound scan and renal biopsy. What chromosomal abnormality is most likely associated with the development of such a tumour?

  a 9

  b 10

  c 11

  d 12

  e 13

55 An eight-year-old girl is referred to the orthopaedic team following pain in her left leg. An X-ray demonstrates evidence of soft tissue calcification and a sunburst-like appearance. What is the most likely diagnosis?

   a Ewing's sarcoma

   b Osteochondroma

   c Osteoid osteoma

   d Osteosarcoma

   e Osteoclastoma

56 A 10-year-old girl is referred to the orthopaedic team following pain and swelling in her right leg. An X-ray demonstrates evidence of an onion skin type appearance. What is the most likely diagnosis?

   a Ewing's sarcoma

   b Osteochondroma

   c Osteoid osteoma

   d Osteosarcoma

   e Osteoclastoma

57 An eight-year-old girl is reviewed by her GP. On examination the GP notes evidence of skin erythema, with vesicles and papules on her face, extensor and flexor surfaces of her arms and legs. Her mother states that she is always scratching her skin. What is the most likely diagnosis?

   a Eczema

   b Seborrhoeic dermatitis

   c Psoriasis

   d Pityriasis rosea

   e Erythema multiforme

58 A two-month-old boy is brought to the GP by his mother. His mother has noticed a thick yellow scale on his scalp as well as redness and scaling of both his arms. What is the most likely diagnosis?

a Eczema

b Seborrhoeic dermatitis

c Psoriasis

d Pityriasis rosea

e Erythema multiforme

59 A seven-year-old boy is reviewed by his GP. On examination the GP notes evidence of silvery grey plaques on the extensor surfaces of his elbows. What is the most likely diagnosis?

a Eczema

b Seborrhoeic dermatitis

c Psoriasis

d Pityriasis rosea

e Erythema multiforme

60 An 11-year-old boy is reviewed by his GP. On examination the GP notes the presence of rose pink macules on his trunk in the distribution of a Christmas tree. What is the most likely diagnosis?

a Eczema

b Seborrhoeic dermatitis

c Psoriasis

d Pityriasis rosea

e Erythema multiforme

61 A young boy is recently diagnosed with erythema nodosum. What is the most likely bacterial aetiological cause for this condition?

a *Streptococcus*

b *Haemophilus influenzae*

c *Mycobacterium tuberculosis*

d *Listeria*

e *Legionella*

62 A five-year-old girl is brought to her GP by her mother. On examination the GP notes the presence of yellow crusted lesions on her cheeks. His mother comments it all started with a single red spot on her cheek that looked like a cigarette burn. What is the most likely diagnosis?

a Impetigo

b Erysipelas

c Acne

d Herpes simplex

e Molluscum contagiosum

63 Which investigation is most likely to lead to a diagnosis in the above case?

a Skin swab

b Blood cultures

c Autoantibody screen

d Sputum microscopy and culture

e Urine microscopy and culture

64 A four-year-old boy is recently diagnosed with impetigo. What is the most common aetiological cause for such a condition?

 a *Streptococcus*

 b *Staphylococcus aureus*

 c *Mycobacterium tuberculosis*

 d *Listeria*

 e *Legionella*

65 A young boy is reviewed by his GP. On examination the GP notes a red discolouration of the boy's face with notable swelling. What is the most likely diagnosis?

 a Impetigo

 b Erysipelas

 c Acne

 d Herpes simplex

 e Molluscum contagiosum

66 What is the most likely aetiological cause in the above patient?

 a *Staphylococcus aureus*

 b *Mycobacterium tuberculosis*

 c *Listeria*

 d *Legionella*

 e *Streptococcus*

67 An eight-year-old girl is brought to her GP by her father. Her father is concerned about the development of sores over her mouth. On examination the GP notes evidence of vesicles with crusting in her oral and peri oral region. What is the most likely diagnosis?

a Herpes simplex type 2

b Molluscum contagiosum

c Candida

d Herpes simplex type 1

e Tinea capitis

68 A 10-year-old boy is reviewed by his GP. On general examination the GP notes the presence of flesh-coloured, dome-shaped lesions. What is the most likely diagnosis?

a Herpes simplex type 2

b Molluscum contagiosum

c Candida

d Herpes simplex type 1

e Tinea capitis

69 A nine-year-old girl is recently diagnosed with molluscum contagiosum. What is the most likely aetiological cause for this condition?

a Herpes simplex type 2

b *Staphylococcus*

c *Streptococcus*

d Herpes simplex type 1

e Poxvirus

70 A four-year-old Afro-Caribbean boy is brought to the GP by his father. His father comments that his son's hair is falling out. On examination the GP notes evidence of circumscribed bald patches with scaling. What is the most likely diagnosis?

a Tinea corporis

b Tinea pedis

c Tinea capitis

d Candida

e Scabies

71 A six-year-old boy presents to his GP accompanied by his mother. On examination the GP notes evidence of red patches in his groin and arm pits, which extend to his trunk. What is the most likely diagnosis?

a Tinea capitis

b Tinea corporis

c Tinea pedis

d Scabies

e Erythema nodosum

72 An eight-year-old girl is brought to her GP by her mother. Her mother comments that her daughter has been complaining of itchy feet. On examination the GP notes a white blotting-paper-like appearance of the skin between the girl's toes. What is the most likely diagnosis?

a Tinea capitis

b Tinea corporis

c Tinea pedis

d Scabies

e Erythema nodosum

73 A girl is recently diagnosed with tinea capitis. Which investigation is most likely to lead to a diagnosis?

a Blood cultures

b Full blood count

c Serum liver function tests

d Skin scrapings

e Sputum microscopy and culture

74 An eight-year-old boy presents to the GP with his mother. The GP notes evidence of well-circumscribed bald patches on his scalp. What is the next most appropriate step in management?

a Reassure

b Antidandruff shampoo

c Antiviral agents

d Antifungal agents

e Antibacterial agents

75 A six-year-old girl is brought to her GP by her mother. Her mother comments that her daughter has been scratching her head, face and hands constantly. On examination you note the presence of red papules and vesicles with evidence of crusting. What is the most likely diagnosis?

a Tinea capitis

b Tinea corporis

c Tinea pedis

d Scabies

e Erythema nodosum

76 A girl is suspected to be suffering from scabies. Which investigation is most likely to lead to a diagnosis?

a Blood cultures

b Full blood count

c Serum liver function tests

d Skin scrapings

e Sputum microscopy and culture

77 A two-week-old baby is reviewed by the GP. On examination the GP notes the presence of a raised red-dimple-like lesion on his face. What is the most likely diagnosis?

a Strawberry naevus

b Port wine stain

c Scabies

d Erythema multiforme

e Angiosarcoma

78 The following are all true with regard to a strawberry naevus EXCEPT:

a It affects up to 4% of babies

b It may lead to thrombocytosis

c Treatment may include laser therapy

d Treatment may include cryotherapy

e Treatment may include steroids

79 A newborn baby is reviewed by the GP. On examination the GP notes the presence of flat purple lesions on the baby's face. What is the most likely diagnosis?

a Strawberry nodosum

b Port wine stain

c Scabies

d Erythema multiforme

e Angiosarcoma

80 The following are all true with regards to blood circulation in a newborn baby EXCEPT:

a Pressure in the pulmonary circulation falls

b The pressure in the pulmonary circulation falls over the first six months of life

c The ductus arteriosus closes

d The ductus arteriosus contracts

e There is often a marked increased in blood oxygenation

81 A newborn baby is diagnosed with coarctation of the aorta. The following are all true with regards to coarctation of the aorta EXCEPT:

a The left ventricle may hypertrophy

b Circulation is maintained by the ductus arteriosus

c It may be associated with collapse

d It may result in alkalosis

e It may be associated with pulmonary oedema

82 The following are all true with regards to transposition of the great vessels EXCEPT:

a It is the commonest cause of cyanotic congenital heart disease at birth

b The left ventricle is linked to the pulmonary artery

c Oxygenated blood is delivered to the lungs

d The left ventricle delivers deoxygenated blood to the aorta

e Surgery is the treatment of choice

83 The following are all true with regards to Fallot's tetralogy EXCEPT:

a It is commonly associated with left ventricular hypertrophy

b It is associated with cyanosis

c Surgery is the treatment of choice

d It is commonly associated with right ventricular hypertrophy

e It is associated with pulmonary stenosis

84 A 10-year-old boy is reviewed by the GP. On examination the GP notes a continuous machinery murmur under the left clavicle and a bounding pulse. What is the most likely diagnosis?

a Ventricular septal defect

b Patent ductus arteriosus

c Atrial septal defect

d Aortic stenosis

e Pulmonary stenosis

85 A five-year-old girl is reviewed by the GP. On examination the GP notes an ejection click and a murmur over the aortic area. What is the most likely diagnosis?

a Ventricular septal defect

b Patent ductus arteriosus

c Atrial septal defect

d Aortic stenosis

e Pulmonary stenosis

86 The following are all common causes of sudden cardiac death in childhood EXCEPT:

a Myocarditis

b Pulmonary stenosis

c Hypertrophic obstructive cardiomyopathy

d Prolonged QT syndrome

e Aortic stenosis

87 A mother is concerned about the rate at which her newborn baby is breathing. What is the most likely respiratory rate of a healthy neonate?

a 30–40 breaths per minute

b 20–25 breaths per minute

c 25–30 breaths per minute

d 40–60 breaths per minute

e 60–65 breaths per minute

88   A six-year-old boy is brought to the GP by his mother. He complains of slight discomfort on swallowing. On examination you note the presence of enlarged tonsils covered by a white exudate. What is the most likely aetiological cause for his symptoms?

a   Viral

b   *Streptococcus*

c   *Staphylococcus*

d   *Haemophilus influenzae*

e   *Mycobacterium tuberculosis*

89   A four-year-old boy is brought to the GP by his mother. His mother comments that he has been crying excessively and appears in a lot of pain. General examination reveals the presence of an inflamed tympanic membrane. What is the most likely aetiological cause for his symptoms?

a   *Mycoplasma*

b   *Streptococcus*

c   *Staphylococcus*

d   *Mycobacterium tuberculosis*

e   *Moraxella catarrhalis*

90 A mother of a three-year-old girl telephones her GP for advice about her daughter. She informs the GP that her daughter has been suffering from what she feels is a viral infection but has recently now developed a strong bark-like cough. She says that her daughter looks really exhausted from over-breathing. What is the next most appropriate step in management?

   a Reassure

   b Advise simple paracetamol and rest

   c Advise ibuprofen and rest

   d Advise nil by mouth for 24–48 hours

   e Advise immediate transfer to hospital

91 A three-year-old girl is diagnosed with croup. Her oxygen saturations are 91% on room air. Which management plan would you instigate first?

   a Steroids

   b Salbutamol

   c Atrovent

   d Salbutamol and atrovent

   e Oxygen

92 The following are all true with regards to croup infection EXCEPT:

   a It affects children up to the age of three years

   b It is associated with a bark-like cough

   c It is not associated with swallowing difficulties

   d It is caused by *Haemophilus influenzae* type B

   e It is associated with a viral prodrome

93   A father of a six-year-old Afro-Caribbean boy telephones the GP for
      advice about his son. He comments that his son has been breathing
      in a shallow manner for the past few hours. He goes on to say that
      his son is dribbling from the mouth and appears very unwell. What
      is the most likely diagnosis?

      a Mycobacterium tuberculosis

      b Croup

      c Epiglottitis

      d *Mycoplasma* pneumonia

      e Sarcoidosis

94   What is the next most appropriate step in management for the above
      patient?

      a Rifampicin

      b Steroids

      c Amoxicillin

      d Clarithromycin

      e Ceftriaxone

95   A mother brings her son to A&E. She comments that he has been
      experiencing bouts of coughing, which is associated with him going
      blue. In addition she states that he has been vomiting on occasion.
      Routine blood investigations demonstrate a lymphocyte count of
      60×10^9/L. What is the most likely diagnosis?

      a Mycobacterium tuberculosis

      b Croup

      c Epiglottitis

      d *Mycoplasma* pneumonia

      e Pertussis

96 An eight-month-old girl is brought to A&E. On examination you note evidence of bilateral crepitations in her chest with associated recession and cyanosis. What is the most likely diagnosis?

a Bronchiolitis

b Croup

c Epiglottitis

d Pneumonia

e Pertussis

97 What is the most likely aetiological cause for the above patient's symptoms?

a *Mycobacterium tuberculosis*

b *Mycoplasma pneumoniae*

c *Pneumocystis jiroveci*

d *Haemophilus influenzae* type B

e Respiratory syncytial virus

98 A six-year-old girl with asthma meets the step 4 British Thoracic Society (BTS) criteria of asthma management. What is the most appropriate step in management in this category?

a Short-acting β_2 agonist alone

b Inhaled steroid up to 800 micrograms daily and an inhaled long-acting β_2 agonist

c Long-acting β_2 agonist alone

d Oral prednisolone

e Home nebulisers

99 A three-year-old boy with asthma meets the step 2 BTS criteria of asthma management. What is the most appropriate step in management in this category?

a Short-acting β_2 agonist alone

b Inhaled steroid alone

c Short-acting β_2 agonist and inhaled steroid

d Oral prednisolone

e Home nebulisers

100 A three-year-old boy is seen by his GP. The father comments that his son has been feeling feverish recently and passing urine more frequently than normal. Routine observations reveal a temperature of 39°C. What is the next most appropriate initial investigation?

a MAG 3 scan

b Abdominal ultrasound scan

c MCUG scan

d Urine dip

e Blood cultures

101 A four-year-old boy is reviewed at home by his GP. On examination the GP notes evidence of facial, ankle and abdominal swelling. The boy is otherwise well and appears comfortable. What is the next most appropriate initial investigation?

a Urine dip

b Full blood count

c Abdominal ultrasound scan

d Ankle X-ray

e Continue to observe

102 The following statements are true with regards to infant feeding EXCEPT:

 a Soy milk is recommended between the ages of three and six months

 b Breast-feeding enhances mother–child bonding

 c Breast-feeding is contraindicated in tuberculosis-positive mothers

 d Breast-feeding is contraindicated in HIV-positive mothers

 e Infants with cow's milk allergy should avoid soy milk

103 An 11-week-old baby is brought to A&E. The mother comments that her daughter has been vomiting excessively recently after meals, often in a projectile fashion. What is the most likely diagnosis?

 a Gastro-oesophageal reflux disease

 b Achalasia

 c Gastroenteritis

 d Pyloric stenosis

 e Food allergy

104 An eight-month-old girl is rushed to A&E. On examination she is crying excessively and appears in severe pain. Her mother comments that she has been vomiting recently and has passed red-currant-like stools on occasion. What is the most likely diagnosis?

 a Gastroenteritis

 b Intussusception

 c Appendicitis

 d Ulcerative colitis

 e Crohn's disease

105 An eight-year-old girl is rushed to A&E as a result of feeling unwell at school. Her teacher comments that she had been experiencing central abdominal discomfort and has been vomiting. On examination you note severe tenderness in her epigastric region. Routine observations reveal a pulse of 110 beats per minute and temperature of 39°C. The girl has also been suffering from a chest infection recently. What is the most likely diagnosis?

a Tuberculosis

b Appendicitis

c Mesenteric adenitis

d Pneumonia

e Gastroenteritis

106 A six-year-old boy is witnessed by his teacher at school to complain of feeling funny in his stomach and lip smacking. What is the most likely diagnosis?

a Tonic clonic seizure

b Focal motor seizure

c Temporal lobe seizure

d Drop attack

e Myoclonic jerk

107 The following are all true with regards to cerebral palsy EXCEPT:

a Hemiplegia occurs in approximately 60–65% of all cases of cerebral palsy

b Spastic quadriplegia may be due to birth abnormalities

c Hemiplegia occurs between 16 and 24 months usually

d Cerebral palsy may be linked with learning difficulties

e Cerebral palsy may be linked with seizures

108 A 10-year-old boy is rushed to A&E following a seizure. On general examination you note the presence of depigmented oval patches and leathery patches in the lumbar region. What is the most likely diagnosis?

a Tuberous sclerosis

b Neurofibromatosis type 1

c Neurofibromatosis type 2

d Erythema nodosum

e Scabies

109 Which of the following drugs is specifically associated with congenital heart disease in the fetus?

a Phenytoin

b Warfarin

c Carbamazepine

d Valproate

e Lithium

110 A newborn baby undergoes assessment. On examination you note a heart rate of 80 beats per minute, a regular respiratory effort, well-flexed muscle tone, pink colouration and a grimace when stimulated. What is the most likely Apgar score in this case?

a 2

b 4

c 6

d 8

e 10

111   The following are all true with regards to breast-feeding EXCEPT:

   a   It is associated with a reduced incidence of gastroenteritis

   b   It is associated with an increased risk of necrotising enterocolitis

   c   It is associated with a reduced risk of breast cancer in the mother

   d   It is associated with a reduced risk of osteoporosis in the mother

   e   It is associated with improved cognitive function

112   The following are all true with regards to respiratory distress syndrome EXCEPT:

   a   It is associated with excess surfactant production

   b   It is associated with prematurity

   c   It is associated with an air bronchogram on chest X-ray

   d   It is associated with a ground glass appearance on chest X-ray

   e   It is associated with bilateral pleural effusions on chest X-ray

113   The following are all true with regards to paediatric life support for a six-month-old baby EXCEPT:

   a   Sternal compression should occur with three fingers

   b   Cardiopulmonary resuscitation (CPR) is performed at a ratio of 15:2

   c   If the child is not breathing, five rescue breaths should be given initially

   d   The sternum is compressed at its lower third

   e   One should look, listen and feel for breathing for no more than 10 seconds

114 The following are all true with regards to paediatric life support for a two-year-old child EXCEPT:

a Sternal compression should occur with the heel of one hand

b CPR is performed at a ratio of 15:2

c If the child is not breathing, two rescue breaths should be given initially

d The sternum is compressed at its lower third

e One should look, listen and feel for breathing for no more than 10 seconds

115 A 12-year-old boy is rushed to A&E following concerns raised by his mother. She comments that her son has developed a rash that does not fade on pressure. He is also complaining of a stiff neck and abdominal discomfort. What is the most likely diagnosis?

a Gastroenteritis

b Appendicitis

c Mesenteric adenitis

d Cervical spondylitis

e Meningitis

116 A young boy is reviewed by his GP who notes a short stature, limb shortening and frontal bossing with a flat nasal bride. What is the most likely diagnosis?

a Achondroplasia

b Di George syndrome

c Down's syndrome

d Prader Willi syndrome

e Fragile X syndrome

117 A young boy is reviewed by his GP who notes evidence of gynaeco-mastia and small testes. What is the most likely diagnosis?

a Achondroplasia

b Di George syndrome

c Down's syndrome

d Prader Willi syndrome

e Klinefelter's syndrome

118 A child is reviewed by her GP who notes evidence of blue sclerae and a triangular-shaped face. What is the most likely diagnosis?

a Achondroplasia

b Russell Silver syndrome

c Down's syndrome

d Prader Willi syndrome

e Klinefelter's syndrome

119 A 10-year-old girl is reviewed by her GP who notes evidence of a webbed neck, broad chest and widely spaced nipples. What is the most likely diagnosis?

a Achondroplasia

b Di George syndrome

c Down's syndrome

d Prader Willi syndrome

e Turner's syndrome

120 A two-year-old girl is reviewed by her GP following concerns by her mother. She comments that her daughter seems overweight for her age and continually eats. She goes on to say that she was never like this when she was younger and often had difficulty feeding. What is the most likely diagnosis?

a   Achondroplasia

b   Di George syndrome

c   Down's syndrome

d   Prader Willi syndrome

e   Turner's syndrome

121 The following are all true with regards to attention deficit hyperactivity disorder (ADHD) EXCEPT:

a   It may be associated with a difficulty in concentrating

b   It may be associated with restlessness

c   It is diagnosed by metabolic studies

d   It may be associated with impulsivity

e   It is associated with genetic factors

122 The following are all true with regards to ADHD management EXCEPT:

a   Long chain fatty acids should be avoided

b   Methylphenidate is a useful medication

c   Behavioural therapy may be useful

d   Schizophrenia may be linked to the medical treatment of ADHD

e   Bipolar affective disorder is not associated with the medical treatment of ADHD

123 A four-year-old boy is brought to his GP following concerns raised by his mother. She comments that her son finds it difficult to interact with fellow pupils at school. She also states that he often tends to repeat words and phrases like a parrot and likes to walk on his tip toes. What is the most likely diagnosis?

a Autism

b Down's syndrome

c Asperger's syndrome

d Depression

e ADHD

124 A six-year-old boy is brought to his GP following concerns raised by his father. His father comments that his son finds it difficult to interact with pupils at school and family members. However, he states that his son seems to have a fairly good grasp of the English language. What is the most likely diagnosis?

a Autism

b Down's syndrome

c Asperger's syndrome

d Depression

e ADHD

125 A young boy is brought to A&E complaining of a stiff neck and pain when looking at bright lights. You suspect a diagnosis of meningitis and decide to perform a lumbar puncture. The following are all contraindications to performing a lumbar puncture EXCEPT:

a A serum platelet count of less than $120 \times 10^9/L$

b Respiratory distress

c Shock

d Seizures

e A reduced conscious level

126 A 23-day-old boy is diagnosed with meningitis. What is the most likely aetiological cause for his diagnosis?

a Tuberculosis

b Mumps

c *Streptococcus* group B

d *Meningococcus*

e *Haemophilus influenzae*

127 A 29-day-old boy is diagnosed with meningitis. What is the most likely aetiological cause for his diagnosis?

a Tuberculosis

b Mumps

c *Streptococcus* group B

d *Meningococcus*

e Influenza

128 A neonate is diagnosed with *E. coli* associated meningitis. What is the next most appropriate step in management?

   a Flucloxacillin

   b Fluids

   c Cefotaxime

   d Gentamicin

   e Rifampicin

129 A 30-day-old girl is diagnosed with *Haemophilus influenzae* associated meningitis. What is the next most appropriate step in management?

   a Flucloxacillin

   b Fluids

   c Ceftriaxone

   d Gentamicin

   e Rifampicin

130 A mother telephones her GP following concerns about her daughter. She informs the GP that her daughter has had a temperature of greater than 40°C for the past three days. In addition, she comments that her daughter's temperature has now settled, but she has developed a pale red-spot-like rash on her body, which has spread to her arms and legs. What is the most likely diagnosis?

   a Meningitis

   b Erythema multiforme

   c Measles

   d Erythema nodosum

   e Roseola infantum

131 A young child is rushed to A&E following a fever for more than five days. On examination you note evidence of a maculopapular rash on the child's arms and neck. In addition you note evidence of cervical lymphadenopathy and a strawberry-like tongue. What is the most likely diagnosis?

a Kawasaki's disease

b Scarlet fever

c Meningitis

d Measles

e Herpes simplex

132 A four-year-old boy is reviewed by his GP. On examination the GP notes evidence of white spots on a red coloured background within the boy's mouth. What is the most likely diagnosis?

a Kawasaki's disease

b Scarlet fever

c Meningitis

d Measles

e Herpes simplex

133 A seven-year-old boy is brought to A&E. His mother comments that he has been suffering from a pink coloured maculopapular rash all over his body for the past few days. Prior to that, he had suffered from a cold, which has now settled. What is the most likely diagnosis?

a Kawasaki's disease

b Rubella

c Meningitis

d Measles

e Herpes simplex

134 A 10-year-old boy is rushed to A&E following concerns raised by his mother. The boy has been suffering from a runny nose and fever for the past few days. On general examination you note evidence of a blotchy red-coloured rash on his face, which is non-tender on palpation. What is the most likely diagnosis?

    a Kawasaki's disease

    b Rubella

    c Meningitis

    d Measles

    e Slapped cheek syndrome

135 A young boy is diagnosed with slapped cheek syndrome. What is the most likely aetiological cause of this condition?

    a Parvovirus B12

    b Parvovirus B15

    c Parvovirus B17

    d Parvovirus B19

    e Parvovirus B21

136 A seven-year-old boy is reviewed by his GP. On examination the GP notes evidence of crust covered spots on his abdomen, back, arms and legs. The boy's mother states that the spots were initially small, red and very itchy. What is the most likely diagnosis?

    a Kawasaki's disease

    b Rubella

    c Meningitis

    d Chicken pox

    e Slapped cheek syndrome

137   A 16-year-old boy presents to his GP complaining of a five-day history of a sore throat, fever and aching joints. He is currently in an active relationship. On examination you note evidence of enlarged cervical lymph nodes. You suspect a diagnosis of glandular fever. Which investigation is most likely to lead to a diagnosis?

a   Full blood count

b   Paul Bunnell test

c   HIV test

d   Serum liver function tests

e   Bone profile

138   A young boy is diagnosed with glandular fever following appropriate investigations. What is the most likely aetiological cause of glandular fever?

a   HIV

b   *Mycoplasma pneumoniae*

c   Epstein Barr virus

d   *Haemophilus influenzae*

e   *Streptococcus pneumoniae*

139 An eight-year-old girl is brought to her GP for an urgent assessment. On examination the GP notes evidence of a bright red rash on her neck and chest. In addition, her tongue appears strawberry-like in appearance. Routine observations demonstrate a temperature of 39°C. What is the most likely diagnosis?

a Kawasaki's disease

b Rubella

c Meningitis

d Chicken pox

e Scarlet fever

140 What is the next most appropriate step in management for the above patient?

a Fluids

b Paracetamol

c Reassure

d Penicillin

e Rifampicin

141 The following are all true with regards to blood sampling in children EXCEPT:

a One should use lidocaine intramuscularly prior to the procedure

b A butterfly needle is preferred

c Alcohol swabs should be utilised

d Vacuum systems are often not tolerated by children

e Non-sterile gloves should be worn

142 The following are all true with regards to cannulation in children EXCEPT:

  a Preferred sites include the antecubital fossa

  b Alcohol swabs should be utilised

  c The cannula should be flushed with water or saline

  d Blood may be withdrawn from the cannula

  e Cannulae should be inserted at an angle of 45 degrees

143 The following are all true with regards to intraosseous vascular access in children EXCEPT:

  a It is contraindicated in pelvic fracture

  b The preferred site is three fingers' breadth below and medial to the tibial tuberosity

  c Non-sterile gloves should be used

  d Following the procedure a saline flush should be used

  e Complications may include skin necrosis

144 The following are all true with regards to performing a lumbar puncture in children EXCEPT:

  a It is contraindicated if the platelet count is less than $100 \times 10^9/L$

  b It is contraindicated if there are signs of raised intracranial pressure

  c It is contraindicated if there evidence of a reduced level of consciousness

  d The ideal landmark is between L3 and L4

  e At least six drops of cerebrospinal fluid (CSF) should be obtained for each sample pot

145 The following are all true with regards to suprapubic aspiration of urine in children EXCEPT:

a A 14 G needle is preferred

b The procedure involves an aseptic technique

c Alcohol swabs are essential

d The perineum should ideally be cleaned first

e The landmark point is approximately one finger's breadth above the symphysis pubis

146 The following are all true with regards to chest drain insertion in children EXCEPT:

a A chest X-ray should be performed after insertion

b In neonates the treatment of a tension pneumothorax involves insertion of a cannula in the 4th intercostal space mid-clavicular line

c The procedure requires a full aseptic technique

d Local anaesthetic should be infiltrated with an orange needle

e Full monitoring of oxygen saturation and pulse rate is required

147 The following are all true with regards to endotracheal intubation in children EXCEPT:

a Oxygen saturation and heart rate should be monitored throughout

b Pre-oxygenation is often required

c Neonates should maintain a neutral head position

d Premature infants often require a 6.0 tube size

e The laryngoscope should ideally be held in the left hand

148 The following are all true with regards to radial arterial cannulation in children EXCEPT:

a The wrist should be slightly extended

b Firm pressure should be applied for at least five minutes post-procedure

c There is a risk of arterial spasm

d Gloves should be worn

e An angle higher than that used in venous cannulation should be observed

149 The following are all true with regards to umbilical arterial catheter insertion EXCEPT:

a One should aim to insert the catheter tip below L1 in the low position

b An aseptic technique is required

c Arterial spasm may occur

d Anaesthetic is not required

e The umbilical artery catheter depth equates to the weight (kg) × 3 + 9 cm

150 The following are all true with regards to umbilical venous catheter insertion EXCEPT:

a The position of the line should be checked with a chest and abdominal X-ray

b An aseptic technique is required

c Arterial spasm may occur

d Anaesthetic is not required

e The umbilical venous catheter depth equates to the weight (kg) × 3 + 6 cm

151 The following are all true with regards to Mongolian blue spots EXCEPT:

   a They are common among dark-skinned individuals

   b They may increase one's risk of cancer

   c They are usually 2–8 cm in width

   d They usually present as blue or blue grey-coloured lesions

   e They may be irregular in shape

152 The following are all causes of neonatal jaundice in those less than 24 hours of age EXCEPT:

   a ABO incompatibility

   b G6PD deficiency

   c Spherocytosis

   d Rhesus incompatibility

   e Biliary atresia

153 The following are all true with regards to Group B *Streptococcus* infection EXCEPT:

   a Neonatal infection rate is often low

   b Prematurity is a risk factor for transmission

   c Prolonged membrane rupture is a risk factor for transmission

   d Maternal intrapartum fever is a risk factor for transmission

   e Rifampicin is the treatment of choice

154 The following statements are all true with regards to periventricular haemorrhage in children EXCEPT:

a Premature infants have an increased risk of haemorrhage

b Infants greater than 32 weeks gestation have an increased risk of haemorrhage

c Hypoxia is a risk factor

d Hypotension is a risk factor

e Grade III haemorrhage is associated with an increased risk of cerebral palsy

155 A child is born with a cleft lip. The following are all true with regards to cleft lip formation EXCEPT:

a It may be diagnosed by ultrasound in the second trimester

b It is due to failure of merging of the medial nasal and maxillary processes at 10 weeks gestation

c It may be associated with a cleft palate

d It may be associated with feeding difficulties

e The *TGFB3* gene may be associated with the formation of cleft lip

156 A four-year-old girl is reviewed by her GP. On examination the GP notes the presence of a white left pupil, which does not react to light. What is the most likely diagnosis?

a Retinoblastoma

b Conjunctivitis

c Glaucoma

d Orbital cellulitis

e Iritis

157 A 10-year-old boy is brought to his GP. On examination the GP notes evidence of redness of his right eye. The boy's mother comments that she has noted evidence of crusting and a purulent discharge on occasion. What is the most likely diagnosis?

a Retinoblastoma

b Conjunctivitis

c Glaucoma

d Orbital cellulitis

e Iritis

158 A four-year-old boy is reviewed by his GP. On general examination the GP notes evidence of lacrimation and excessive blinking of his right eye. In addition the boy's mother comments that her son is having difficulty looking at bright lights. What is the most likely diagnosis?

a Retinoblastoma

b Conjunctivitis

c Glaucoma

d Orbital cellulitis

e Iritis

159 A five-year-old boy undergoes a routine eye assessment. Slit lamp examination reveals the presence of an irregular right pupil. In addition, the anterior chamber appears excessively cloudy. What is the most likely diagnosis?

a Retinoblastoma

b Conjunctivitis

c Glaucoma

d Orbital cellulitis

e Iritis

160 A six-year-old boy is brought to A&E by his mother. On examination you note evidence of erythema around his right eye. In addition, you note evidence of right-sided proptosis and reduced eye movements. What is the most likely diagnosis?

a Retinoblastoma

b Conjunctivitis

c Glaucoma

d Orbital cellulitis

e Iritis

Extended matching questions

Theme: Immunisation

a 1 month

b 2 months

c 3 months

d 4 months

e 12 months

f 3 years

g 13 months

h Birth

i 6 months

j 7 months

For each scenario described below, choose the single most appropriate answer from the above list of options. Each option may be used once, more than once or not at all.

1   The hepatitis B vaccine is given at this time to all babies born to hepatitis-B-positive mothers.

2   The Bacillus Calmette-Guérin (BCG) vaccine is given at this time to all babies who are born in a tuberculosis-prevalent area.

3   The *Haemophilus influenzae* type B and *meningococcus C* vaccine are only given together at this age.

4   The measles, mumps and rubella (MMR) and pneumococcal vaccine together are only given at this age.

5   The first *Haemophilus influenzae* type B vaccine is given at this time.

Theme: Respiratory conditions

a Tuberculosis

b Croup

c Pertussis

d *Mycoplasma* pneumonia

e Epiglottitis

f Asthma

g Bronchiolitis

h Cystic fibrosis

i *Legionella* pneumonia

j Bronchiectasis

For each scenario described below, choose the single most appropriate answer from the above list of options. Each option may be used once, more than once or not at all.

1   Associated with a severe bark-like cough.

2   Associated with bouts of coughing, which may result in subsequent bronchopneumonia.

3   Known to cause significant dysphagia in the absence of a cough.

4   Commonly seen in children under the age of one year with evidence of crepitations, chest recession and cyanosis.

5   A young girl who experiences significant wheezing and breathlessness mainly at night and first thing in the morning. It is often made worse by exercise and cold weather.

Theme: Rashes

a Meningitis

b Measles

c Rubella

d Roseola infantum

e Chicken pox

f Erythema multiforme

g Erythema nodosum

h Eczema

i Urticaria

j Henoch Schonlein purpura

For each scenario described below, choose the single most appropriate answer from the above list of options. Each option may be used once, more than once or not at all.

1 Associated with a fever and red-coloured papules, which eventually develop into crusted vesicles.

2 Caused by the human herpes virus 6B.

3 Associated initially with the presence of white salt-like spots inside the mouth.

4 A worrying illness associated with fever, neck stiffness and a non-blanching rash.

5 Large red-blotch-like lesions seen following the consumption of shellfish, which improve with antihistamine medication.

Theme: Skin disorders

a Eczema

b Seborrhoeic dermatitis

c Psoriasis

d Pityriasis rosea

e Urticaria

f Erythema nodosum

g Impetigo

h Cellulitis

i Molluscum contagiosum

j Scabies

For each scenario described below, choose the single most appropriate answer from the above list of options. Each option may be used once, more than once or not at all.

1 Associated with an erythematous, papular rash affecting the flexural and extensor surfaces of the arms and legs.

2 A disorder known to affect children in the first three months of life and associated with a thick yellow scale on their scalp.

3 A viral disorder known to produce rose pink-coloured lesions in the distribution of a Christmas tree on the trunk.

4 A disorder associated with large red-coloured lesions on the shins in children with Crohn's disease.

5 A disorder associated with the development of red vesicular spots on the face, which subsequently develop into gold-coloured crusts.

Theme: Epileptic seizures

a Tonic clonic

b Focal motor

c Temporal lobe

d Myoclonic jerk

e Absence

f Drop attack

g West's syndrome

h Rolandic

i Lennox Gastaut syndrome

j Landau Kleffner syndrome

For each scenario described below, choose the single most appropriate answer from the above list of options. Each option may be used once, more than once or not at all.

1 Associated with difficulties in understanding and speaking words.

2 Characterised by sudden stiffness and irregular jerk-like movements.

3 Associated with lip smacking and an unusual sensation in the stomach.

4 A form of epilepsy that may be seen in children with tuberous sclerosis.

5 Common in the first year of life and associated with flexion spasms typically every 10 seconds.

Theme: Genetic disorders

a   Achondroplasia

b   Prader Willi syndrome

c   Marfan's syndrome

d   Fragile X syndrome

e   Klinefelter's syndrome

f   Trisomy 13

g   Trisomy 18

h   Turner's syndrome

i   William's syndrome

j   Russell Silver syndrome

For each scenario described below, choose the single most appropriate answer from the above list of options. Each option may be used once, more than once or not at all.

1   A condition associated with a small stature and blue sclerae.

2   Known to cause congenital heart disease in the vast majority of cases. Presents with a small mouth and low-set ears.

3   Seen in females and associated with a short stature and a webbed neck.

4   A genetic disorder caused by the deletion of genetic material from the region q11.23 of chromosome 7.

5   A genetic disorder associated with a cleft lip and rocker bottom feet.

Theme: Developmental milestones

a 3–6 months

b 16–24 months

c 1 month

d 10–18 months

e Birth

f 8 months

g 14 months–2 years

h 3 years

i 4 years

j 6–10 months

For each scenario described below, choose the single most appropriate answer from the above list of options. Each option may be used once, more than once or not at all.

1 Demonstration of a palmar grasp.

2 Demonstration of a pincer grasp.

3 Holding a spoon and transferring food into the mouth.

4 Demonstration of polysyllabic babbling.

5 Building a tower of three to four bricks.

Theme: The Apgar score

a 1

b 2

c 3

d 4

e 5

f 6

g 7

h 8

i 9

j 0

For each scenario described below, choose the single most appropriate answer from the above list of options. Each option may be used once, more than once or not at all.

1   Pink extremities, a pulse rate of 120 beats per minute, a cough when stimulated, some flexion and strong breathing.

2   Cyanosed, a pulse rate of 60 beats per minute, a grimace when stimulated, active movement and weak breathing.

3   A pink body with blue extremities, a pulse rate of 80 beats per minute, a grimace when stimulated, active movement and strong breathing.

4   Cyanosis, no pulse, no stimulation response, some flexion, absent breathing.

5   Cyanosis, no pulse, no stimulation response, no flexion, absent breathing.

Theme: Tumours

a Hodgkin's lymphoma

b Non-Hodgkin's lymphoma

c Wilm's tumour

d Glioma

e Medulloblastoma

f Neuroblastoma

g Osteosarcoma

h Ewing's sarcoma

i Craniopharyngioma

j Acute myeloid leukaemia

For each scenario described below, choose the single most appropriate answer from the above list of options. Each option may be used once, more than once or not at all.

1 Associated with firm painless lymph node swellings and the presence of Reed-Sternberg cells on histology.

2 Associated with jerky eye movements and small blue-coloured lumps in the skin.

3 A condition associated with haematuria and an abdominal mass.

4 Associated with a painful limp and a sunburst-like appearance on limb X-ray.

5 Arises from astrocytes and accounts for over 50% of all childhood brain tumours.

Theme: Cardiology

a Ventricular septal defect

b Pulmonary stenosis

c Mitral stenosis

d Atrial septal defect

e Mitral regurgitation

f Aortic stenosis

g Patent ductus arteriosus

h Tetralogy of Fallot

i Coarctation of the aorta

j Pulmonary stenosis

For each scenario described below, choose the single most appropriate answer from the above list of options. Each option may be used once, more than once or not at all.

1 Associated with a harsh pansystolic murmur and splitting of the second heart sound.

2 Associated with a loud continuous machinery murmur.

3 Associated with a slow rising pulse and ejection systolic murmur at the apex.

4 Known to cause a systolic murmur in the pulmonary area with fixed splitting of the second heart sound.

5 Associated with an ejection systolic murmur and delayed femoral pulses.

Answers

Single best answer

1 e

A palmar grasp is more commonly observed from the age of six months.

2 d

The primitive reflexes include the grasp, moro, rooting and walking reflex.

3 e

Crawling is most commonly seen between the ages of 9 and 15 months.

4 b

Walking in children is most commonly seen from 18 months onwards.

5 c

Jumping is typically seen between the ages of 36 and 48 months.

6 b

Hand dominance occurs between 18 and 30 months usually.

7   a

Babbling is initially seen between 6 and 12 months.

8   b

Dyspraxia is associated with a difficulty in performing motor-related or verbal tasks. It is seen more commonly in boys than girls.

9   a

In suspected cases of nocturnal enuresis, a urine dipstick is essential to ensure no evidence of infection.

10   e

A star chart is the initial form of management to help encourage children to have a dry night. If this fails, treatments such as alarms or desmopressin may be useful.

11   d

This is most definitely an alarming case and points towards non-accidental injury. Once social services are aware, a case conference is held to assess whether the child should be placed on a child protection register.

12   b

This condition is more common in boys than girls and is often bilateral. Treatment typically involves physiotherapy and splinting.

13   c

Also known as bow legs, this condition is common in those aged less than three years.

14   d

Also known as knock knees, this condition typically affects children between the ages of two and six.

15   d

Pes planus or flat feet is classically a painless condition and is improved by utilisation of arch supports.

16   a

This condition classically follows a viral infection. It is often associated with decreased internal rotation of the hip.

17   a

NSAIDs are the gold standard treatment choice for this condition.

18   c

The condition typically presents with a limp and pain referred to the thigh or knee.

19   b

This condition is associated with necrosis of the capital femoral epiphysis. It is more common in boys and is often bilateral. Over time there is evidence of fragmentation and reossification within the femoral epiphysis.

20   d

Traction allows for the femoral head to be maintained within the acetabulum.

21   c

The condition is often bilateral in 35% of cases and is treated surgically.

22   b

X-ray findings demonstrate a posterior and inferior slip of the epi-physis on the metaphysis. Lateral X-ray views are essential.

23   d

This test is known as the Barlow's test. An alternative screening test is the Ortolani manoeuvre. Developmental dysplasia of the hip is much more common in girls and is always looked for at birth.

24   a

An ultrasound scan is the gold standard diagnostic test for develop-mental dysplasia of the hip.

25   e

Septic arthritis is commonly caused by *Staphylococcus* or *Streptococcus* species and can lead to destruction of the articular cartilage and bone.

26   c

Classical presentation of osteomyelitis. The most common sites of infection include the metaphysis of the distal femur or proximal tibia.

27   a

Additional organisms include *Streptococcus* and *Haemophilus influenzae*.

28   a

As most cases of osteomyelitis are due to *Staphylococcus* species, flu-cloxacillin would be the treatment of choice.

29 c

Hot spots are also classical findings but are only seen following a bone scan and not an X-ray.

30 e

In this case the boy has unfortunately developed septic arthritis of the knee, most likely due to infection spreading from his previous osteomyelitis.

31 d

This is a case of juvenile idiopathic arthritis. The first-line treatment of such a condition is NSAIDs.

32 d

This condition is classically associated with a preceding upper respiratory tract infection as in the case described. Gastrointestinal bleeding is common and hence the appearance of melaena. Additional symptoms include abdominal pain and joint discomfort.

33 a

Jaundice in a newborn baby is most commonly due to haemolysis. Phototherapy is the first-line treatment followed by exchange transfusion if this fails to be of benefit.

34 b

Thalassemia is associated with gene deletion resulting in reduced synthesis of alpha or beta globin chains. Following the use of supravital stain, inclusions are seen within red blood cells, which precipitate to give a golf-ball-like appearance. Such inclusions are termed Heinz bodies.

35 c

Beta thalassemia is associated with skeletal abnormalities such as frontal bossing.

36 a

Haemophilia A is due to a deficiency of factor VIII and hence replacement of this factor is the mainstay form of treatment.

37 c

Autoimmune thrombocytopenic purpura in children is often seen following a viral infection. Blood investigations often show evidence of thrombocytopenia with increased megakaryocytes.

38 e

Platelet transfusion or immunoglobulins are the mainstay form of treatment.

39 b

Also known as Christmas disease, this condition arises from a deficiency in factor IX and hence its replacement is the most appropriate management step.

40 d

Von Willebrand's disease is always associated with prolongation of APTT and bleeding times. Platelet count may be reduced but is often normal.

41 a

In addition to von Willebrand factor, factor VIII is also deficient in this disease.

42   d

Desmopressin enables an immediate increase in von Willebrand factor and factor VIII levels.

43   a

Aplastic anaemia is simply a deficiency of all haematopoietic cells. As a result, people are more prone to bleeding and risk of infection as in the case described.

44   a

Bone marrow aspiration is the gold standard diagnostic investigation in aplastic anaemia.

45   d

Blast cells are characteristic of acute leukaemia.

46   a

Hyperkalaemia is a consequence of acute tumour lysis syndrome.

47   a

Cervical lymphadenopathy is common in children. Unilateral lymphadenopathy, as in this case, is often due to *Staphylococcus* or *Streptococcus* species.

48   b

Classic presentation of Hodgkin's lymphoma. Reed-Sternberg cells are the typical histological appearances seen following biopsy and histology.

49   b

The mainstay form of treatment is chemotherapy or radiotherapy.

50   e

Treatment of such a tumour is typically with surgery and radiotherapy.

51   c

The presence of jerk like eye movements is characteristic of a neuroblastoma, often referred to as dancing eyes.

52   a

Neuroblastoma arises from the adrenal glands or sympathetic nerve roots. It subsequently releases catecholamines which can be measured in the urine.

53   b

An abdominal mass is commonly seen in those with a neuroblastoma and may cause abdominal pain and vomiting.

54   c

Abnormalities of chromosome 11 result in an increased risk of Wilm's tumour.

55   d

X-ray findings of a sunburst appearance are characteristic of an osteosarcoma.

56   a

An onion skin type appearance on X-ray is characteristic of an Ewing's sarcoma.

57 a

Classical description of eczema which typically affects flexor and extensor limb surfaces. Treatment involves the use of emollients, anti-inflammatory agents and antihistamines.

58 b

A thick yellow scalp is characteristic of seborrhoeic dermatitis in children. Treatment typically involves olive oil or antifungal shampoos.

59 c

Classical presentation of psoriasis. Treatment typically involves vitamin D analogues or steroid preparations.

60 d

The Christmas tree distribution is characteristic of pityriasis rosea. The condition is notably itchy and this may be improved with aqueous cream.

61 a

Erythema nodosum typically presents as large red patches over the shins. Additional organisms include *Mycoplasma* and *Mycobacterium tuberculosis*.

62 a

Classical presentation of impetigo. It initially presents as red spots, which then develop a yellow crust.

63 a

A skin swab is the most appropriate diagnostic test for impetigo.

64 b

Additional organisms include *Streptococcus*.

65 b

In addition, the condition may result in fever and pain. Treatment is typically with antibiotic therapy.

66 e

The condition is classically due to group A and non-group A *Streptococcus* species.

67 d

Treatment typically involves the use of topical or oral acyclovir.

68 b

The condition usually resolves by itself after six to eight weeks. Treatment typically involves the use of cryotherapy or iodine solution.

69 b

Poxvirus is classically associated with the development of molluscum contagiosum.

70 c

Classical presentation of tinea capitis. The use of UV light demonstrates the presence of green fluorescence, which is diagnostic of tinea capitis.

71 b

Classical presentation of tinea corporis, also known as ringworm. Treatment typically involves the use of topical imidazoles.

72   c

The condition is diagnosed by skin or nail clippings and may be treated through the use of topical imidazoles.

73   d

Skin scrapings are the gold standard diagnostic investigation for tinea capitis.

74   d

This patient has tinea capitis. Treatment involves the use of antifungal agents.

75   d

Scabies is caused by the mite *Sarcoptes scabiei*. Treatment typically involves the use of malathion solution.

76   d

Microscopic analysis of skin scrapings is the gold standard diagnostic test.

77   a

Strawberry naevus is common in preterm infants. Treatment may involve the use of laser or cryotherapy. Additional treatments include the use of steroids and interferon.

78   b

Thrombocytopenia and subsequent bleeding is common in those with strawberry naevus.

79   b

In certain cases, the presence of such lesions on the upper cheek and forehead may be associated with an intracranial vascular malformation with subsequent epilepsy, a condition known as Sturge-Weber syndrome.

80   b

The pulmonary pressure tends to drop over the first one to two months of life.

81   d

Coarctation of the aorta tends to result in acidosis. This is commonly seen in severe cases of coarctation due to circulatory shock with resulting renal impairment and hence impaired excretion of hydrogen ions.

82   b

In transposition of the great vessels, the left ventricle delivers oxygenated blood through the pulmonary artery to the lungs.

83   a

Fallot's tetralogy is associated with right ventricular hypertrophy.

84   b

Patent ductus arteriosus may result in pulmonary hypertension and hence urgent treatment is necessary.

85   d

The murmur of aortic stenosis may be transmitted to the neck.

86 b

Aortic stenosis is more commonly associated with sudden cardiac death in children.

87 d

40–60 breaths per minute for a neonate is deemed a normal respiratory rate.

88 a

This is tonsillitis and the vast majority of tonsillitis is viral in children.

89 b

This child has otitis media. The most likely aetiological cause of otitis media is *Streptococcus*.

90 e

This child has croup in view of her barking cough and previous viral infection. Hospital admission is necessary and treatment with steroids is essential.

91 e

Steroids and bronchodilators are useful treatments for croup. However in this case the patient has significantly low oxygen saturations and therefore high flow oxygen would be the initial treatment of choice. As a useful note, whenever faced with an acute situation always remember the universal 'ABC' approach.

92 d

Croup is caused by the parainfluenza virus.

93   c

This boy has characteristic features of epiglottitis. This condition typically affects children between the ages of three and seven years and occurs within hours. There is often no associated cough.

94   e

Third generation cephalosporins such as ceftriaxone are the most useful treatments of choice.

95   e

This condition is caused by *Bordetella pertussis*. The coughing bouts are due to severe necrosis within the pulmonary epithelium. Pneumonia and seizures may be associated with the condition.

96   a

A condition common in children under the age of one year. Treatment involves the use of oxygen and bronchodilators.

97   e

Respiratory syncytial virus is the most common cause of bronchiolitis.

98   b

For further information regarding asthma management please refer to the British Thoracic Society guidelines, available at: www.brit-thoracic.org.uk

99   c

For further information regarding asthma management please refer to the British Thoracic Society guidelines, available at: www.brit-thoracic.org.uk

100   d

This boy is most likely to be suffering from a urinary tract infection. A urine dipstick is therefore the first line investigation for the condition.

101   a

Classical presentation of nephrotic syndrome, a condition associated with oedema, proteinuria and hypoalbuminemia.

102   a

Soy milk is not recommended under the age of six months due to excessive plant oestrogens and subsequent infertility risks.

103   d

Projectile vomiting is characteristic of pyloric stenosis. Gastric peristalsis is often visible through the wall of the abdomen. Treatment involves surgical division of the pyloric muscle known as a Ramstedt's pyloromyotomy.

104   b

Intussusception is associated with redcurrant-like stools due to subsequent bowel ischaemia. Treatment involves a contrast-based enema or surgery.

105   c

This could be mistaken for appendicitis. However the clue here lies in the fact that the girl had suffered from a recent chest infection. Mesenteric adenitis tends to be associated with upper respiratory tract infections.

106 c

Additional signs may include mouthing or repetitive hand movements.

107 c

Hemiplegia tends to present between 6 and 10 months of age.

108 a

The oval patches are commonly referred to as ash leaf macules. The patches, which are more leathery in nature, are known as shagreen patches.

109 e

Lithium is classically associated with congenital heart disease in the fetus.

110 d

The Apgar score comprises skin complexion, pulse rate, reflex irritability, muscle tone and breathing rate. A score between 7 and 10 is deemed normal.

111 b

Breast-feeding in fact is associated with a lower risk of necrotising enterocolitis.

112 a

Respiratory distress syndrome is in fact associated with reduced surfactant production. Surfactant is a lipoprotein mixture produced by type II pneumocytes and helps to lower surface tension.

113   a

Sternal compression in this age group should occur with two fingers.

114   c

In paediatric basic life support five rescue breaths should be given initially. See Figure 1.

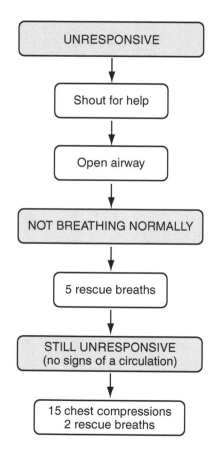

After 1 minute call resuscitation team then continue CPR

Figure 1: Paediatric Basic Life Support Algorithm. Available from: www.resus.org.uk

115   e

A worrying case with some key features of meningitis. An additional worrying symptom would be photophobia.

116   a

Classical presentation of achondroplasia. This is an autosomal dominant condition associated with growth, movement and hearing abnormalities.

117   e

Individuals with this condition are likely to suffer from infertility and learning difficulties.

118   b

Additional features include short stature, micrognathia and hemi-hypertrophy.

119   e

Classical presentation of Turner's syndrome. Individuals with this condition suffer from a reduced life expectancy due to an increased risk of cardiovascular disease.

120   d

Prader Willi syndrome is associated with a defect on chromosome 15. Initially it is associated with poor feeding, due to an impaired swallowing reflex, which then eventually progresses to hyperphagia.

121   c

ADHD is a clinical diagnosis. There are no current diagnostic tests for the condition.

122   e

Bipolar affective disorder is in fact associated in individuals following medical treatment of ADHD.

123   a

Autism is characterised by impaired social functioning, impaired communication, repetitive behaviours and stereotyped movements. Boys tend to be more affected than girls.

124   c

Asperger's syndrome is characterised by social impairments without evidence of significantly impaired language.

125   a

A platelet count of less than 50×10^9/L is a contraindication to a lumbar puncture.

126   c

Additional organisms at this age include *E. coli* and *Listeria*.

127   d

Additional organisms at this age include *Meningococcus*, *Haemophilus influenzae* and *Pneumococcus*.

128   c

Alternative treatment regimens include the use of ampicillin and gentamicin.

129 c

This treatment is also suitable for *Haemophilus influenzae* and *Pneumococcus*-associated meningitis.

130 e

Roseola infantum classically presents with a rose pink rash and fever. Febrile convulsions are common. The rash classically appears following a drop in core body temperature. The condition is caused by the human herpes virus 6B.

131 a

Classical presentation of Kawasaki's disease. All children should have an urgent echo due to the risk of developing coronary artery aneurysms.

132 d

Such spots are known as Koplik's spots. They are a precursor to the development of a rash which is maculopapular in nature.

133 b

Additional symptoms include painful eye movements.

134 e

Classical presentation of slapped cheek syndrome.

135 d

Parvovirus B19 is the major aetiological cause of slapped cheek syndrome.

136   d

Chicken pox is caused by varicella zoster. In certain cases there may be inflammation of the cerebellum resulting in subsequent ataxia.

137   b

It is important to note that antibiotics such as amoxicillin should be avoided in those with glandular fever as it predisposes to a maculopapular rash.

138   c

Epstein Barr virus is the primary cause of glandular fever.

139   e

Classic presentation of scarlet fever. The major cause of the condition is beta haemolytic *Streptococcus*.

140   d

The treatment of choice in those with scarlet fever.

141   a

Lidocaine topically should be applied prior to the procedure and not intramuscularly. It takes approximately 40 minutes to 1 hour to work.

142   c

Cannulae should only be flushed with 0.9% saline and never water.

143   b

With regards to intraosseous access, the preferred site is one finger's breadth below and medial to the tibial tuberosity.

144   a

Lumbar punctures are contraindicated if the platelet count is less than $50 \times 10^9/L$.

145   a

For suprapubic urine aspiration a 21 G needle is preferred.

146   b

A tension pneumothorax is treated by needle insertion into the second intercostal space mid clavicular line.

147   d

For premature infants a 3.0 or 2.5 tube size is required. Tube size is generally calculated with the formula age/4 + 4.

148   e

An angle lower than that used in venous cannulation should be utilised.

149   a

For umbilical arterial catheter insertion, the catheter tip should be inserted below L4 in the low position and above T10 in the high position.

150   e

The umbilical venous catheter depth equates to the weight (kg) × 3 + 9 cm.

151   b

There is no associated cancer risk with Mongolian blue spots. They require no treatment and resolve spontaneously.

152   e

Biliary atresia is a cause of neonatal jaundice in those greater than two weeks of age.

153   e

The preferred treatment of choice is a penicillin or cephalosporin with an aminoglycoside.

154   b

Infants greater than 32 weeks gestation have a reduced risk of haemorrhage.

155   b

Cleft lip formation is due to failure of medial nasal and maxillary processes at five weeks gestation.

156   a

Classical presentation of a retinoblastoma. This is a tumour of photoreceptor cells and is often associated with gene deletion on chromosome 13. Treatment involves cryotherapy or radiotherapy.

157   b

Classical features of conjunctivitis. Most conjunctivitis cases are viral and treatment involves salt water bathing. However, the case described is bacterial in nature and would require topical chloramphenicol eye drops.

158   c

The excessive blinking described is known as blepharospasm. Treatment is often surgical.

159   e

Classical presentation of iritis. Treatment requires antibiotics. Complications include glaucoma and cataract formation.

160   d

Classical presentation of orbital cellulitis. Intravenous antibiotics are often essential as well as an urgent orbital CT scan to exclude sinister pathology.

Extended matching questions

Theme: Immunisation

1 h

2 h

3 e

4 g

5 b

When to immunise	Diseases protected against	Vaccine given
Two months old	Diphtheria, tetanus, pertussis (whooping cough), polio and *Haemophilus influenzae* type B (Hib) pneumococcal infection	DTaP/IPV/Hib and pneumococcal conjugate vaccine (PCV)
Three months old	Diphtheria, tetanus, pertussis, polio and Hib, Meningitis C (meningococcal group C) (MenC)	DTaP/IPV/Hib and MenC
Four months old	Diphtheria, tetanus, pertussis, polio and Hib, MenC, pneumococcal infection	DTaP/IPV/Hib and MenC and PCV
Around 12 months	Hib and MenC	Hib/MenC
Around 13 months	Measles, mumps and rubella (German measles) (MMR), pneumococcal infection	MMR and PCV
Three years and four months or soon after	Diphtheria, tetanus, pertussis and polio, MMR	DTaP/IPV or dTaP/IPV and MMR
Girls aged 12–13 years	Cervical cancer caused by human papillomavirus types 16 and 18	HPV
13–18 years old	Tetanus, diphtheria and polio	Td/IPV

Available from: www.immunisation.nhs.uk

Theme: Respiratory conditions

1   b Croup commonly affects children between the ages of six
        months and three years. It is caused by the parainfluenza
        virus and is best treated with steroids.

2   c Pertussis is caused by *Bordatella pertussis*. In many cases,
        children may develop cyanosis as they are unable to catch
        their breath. Treatment is based on antibiotic therapy.

3   e This condition is due to *Haemophilus influenzae* type B.
        Children are often acutely unwell and treatment is typically
        with the use of ceftriaxone.

4   g Bronchiolitis is caused by the respiratory syncytial virus.
        Treatment is with oxygen and bronchodilator therapy.

5   f Classical presentation of asthma.

Theme: Rashes

1   e Chicken pox is caused by varicella zoster. In certain cases there may be cerebellar inflammation and subsequent ataxia.

2   d This condition is characterised by the presence of a rose pink rash. Treatment is with antibiotics.

3   b Such spots are referred to as Koplik spots and often appear before the presence of the rash associated with measles.

4   a Classic presentation of meningitis. Additional symptoms may include a headache or photophobia.

5   i Alternative treatments may include steroid therapy.

Theme: Skin disorders

1   a   Treatment typically involves the use of emollients, anti-inflammatory agents or antihistamine-based preparations.

2   b   This condition is typically seen within the first three months of life. Treatment involves the use of antifungal agents.

3   d   The condition is characteristically itchy and is improved with the use of aqueous cream.

4   f   This condition is also seen in individuals with tuberculosis and sarcoidosis.

5   g   Impetigo is due to *Staphylococcus* or *Streptococcus* species. Diagnosis is primarily by skin swabs.

Theme: Epileptic seizures

1   j Diagnosis is typically by electroencephalogram (EEG).
       Treatment involves the use of sodium valproate and
       ethosuximide.

2   a Classical description of a tonic clonic seizure. Additional
       features may include tongue biting and urinary incontinence.
       Those affected by such seizures tend to be significantly
       sleepy and confused following the event.

3   c Individuals may also experience possible déjà vu or jamais vu
       in addition to unusual sensory phenomenon.

4   i Such a condition is diagnosed by EEG. Treatment in this
       case is complex and may require an array of antiepileptic
       medications.

5   g Treatment of such a condition is primarily with vigabatrin.

Theme: Genetic disorders

1   j Additional features include a triangular face and hemihypertrophy.

2   g Atrial septal defect, transposition of the great arteries and tetralogy of Fallot are commonly seen.

3   h Associated with a missing X chromosome (45XO). This condition has a reduced life expectancy due to associated cardiovascular disease.

4   i Features include thickened lips, periorbital fullness and a stellate iris.

5   f This condition is associated with a reduced life expectancy due to associated cardiovascular disease.

Theme: Developmental milestones

1   a   Children are also able to transfer objects between their hands
        and can clasp their hands together.

2   d   Children may also be able to hold pencils and scribble at this
        age.

3   g   Hand dominance tends to also appear at this age range.

4   j   At this age children are also able to point to objects they
        want to play with.

5   b   Towers tend to vary in size from three to eight bricks in
        height.

Theme: The Apgar score

1   i

2   e

3   g

4   a

5   j

The Apgar score is comprised of five criteria: appearance, pulse rate, reflex irritability, muscle tone and respiratory rate. A score of 7–10 is deemed normal. Please refer to Finster M, Wood M. The Apgar score has survived the test of time. *Anesthesiology.* 2005; **102**(4): 855–7, for further information.

Theme: Tumours

1   a   Reed-Sternberg cells are characteristic of Hodgkin's lymphoma.

2   f   The jerky movements of the eyes in neuroblastoma is often referred to as dancing eyes.

3   c   Such a tumour is linked to genetic defects on chromosome 11.

4   g   Classical radiological findings seen with an osteosarcoma.

5   d   Treatment of gliomas is by chemotherapy and radiotherapy.

Theme: Cardiology

1   a Ventricular septal defect is often associated with the
development of heart failure and may be associated with
subacute bacterial endocarditis.

2   g This murmur is best heard under the left clavicle. Additional
features include a collapsing pulse.

3   f The mainstay form of treatment is valvular dilation. Valvular
replacement is often not required.

4   d Such defects may contribute significantly to the development
of atrial arrhythmias.

5   i Treatment of such a condition is primarily surgical.

Notes

Index

Page numbers to questions (Q) and answers (A) are given in the following format Q/A